Virgin Diet

Lose Weight, Boost your Metabolism and Maintain Healthy Lifestyle

Theresa Bason

Table of Contents

Introduction

The Virgin Diet (VD) is a diet that helps you maintain your desired weight safely and effectively. The diet works by eliminating 7 food groups from your diet that are believed to be the culprits of food intolerance, which ultimately contributes to weight gain and inability to lose weight. These foods should therefore be dropped from the diet to achieve weight-loss goals.

Food intolerance causes inflammation in the body which leads to weight gain and many other health conditions. The Virgin Diet works by encouraging you to eliminate these foods, reintroducing them back to your diet and coming up with a lifetime diet plan that works best for you.

The Virgin Diet is a fast and lasting weight-loss diet. It is transformational, inspirational and effective. You will be able to follow this popular diet with little effort and come up with amazing and delicious home-made recipes that will make your weight-loss journey lot of fun. You may have tried other weight-loss programs and failed to lose weight, despite following your regimen strictly. When you eliminate the 7 food groups from your diet and discover your own food intolerances, you will start to lose weight, look and feel better and you will find it easier to follow the Virgin Diet.

1: What is Virgin Diet?

The Virgin Diet is your solution to food intolerance and weight loss. You should only eat whole natural foods which are unprocessed and avoid genetically modified foods (GMO foods). The foods recommended in this book offer you the nutrients that your body needs while encouraging you to avoid "offending foods" that trigger health problems.

The Virgin Diet is a diet that helps you to lose weight, boost your metabolism and maintain a healthy lifestyle by avoiding food intolerances that you may have. The diet changes are inspirational because of their great effect. Many people believe all natural foods are good for them and that is why many marketers now label almost everything "natural". You should know food intolerance is caused by both natural and artificial foods.

What is the secret to weigh-loss?
The real secret behind weight gain is not what many people think it is. Most people who want to lose weight have been informed that weight gain and obesity is caused by fat, carbs or calories. They are not aware it is caused by food intolerance (FI). When people have intolerance or sensitivity to foods they consume, the food triggers inflammation in the body which leads to weight gain and

development of illnesses and diseases. Food Intolerance causes health conditions such as acne, fatigue, joint problems and gastrointestinal problems, among others. The joint problems include arthritis while gastrointestinal problems include constipation, gas, indigestion and bloating.

The foods that cause food intolerance and sensitivities are referred to as "offending foods" and these are the foods recommended in many weight-loss diet programs. That is why some people try to lose weight following these diet regimens and fail. In fact, there are people who even gain weight despite following the weight-loss programs strictly. This makes them feel frustrated wondering what they did wrong. Many of the foods recommended in some weight-loss programs include low-fat yogurt, diet drinks loaded with artificial sweeteners and egg whites which many people cannot tolerate but they don't realize it. Instead of losing weight, they gain more weight.

These foods are believed to be "healthy" but they have been shown to cause inflammation which triggers weight gain. Take for example artificial sweeteners. They are in fact concentrated sugar which causes weight gain and obesity, even more than sugar itself. This is the same with processed foods and high glycemic index GI foods like potatoes.

The 7 Food Groups

The Virgin Diet encourages you to eliminate the offending foods listed in the 7 food groups to reduce inflammation and relieve symptoms. The foods are then reintroduced to help you create your own lifetime diet which boosts your metabolism and helps you to maintain a healthy lifestyle. The Virgin Diet is very effective and you can lose an average of 7 pounds within the first 7 days by dropping the 7 food groups.

The idea behind this diet is to eliminate the 7 food groups which are:

- Gluten
- Dairy
- Eggs
- Corn
- Soy
- Peanuts
- Sugar and Sweeteners

As we shall see later, each one of these food groups is made up of many types of foods and beverages. Take for example corn, it is found in so many common foods some of which you consume daily.

The Virgin diet is about eliminating the above 7 food groups in Cycle 1 and reintroducing the foods such as dairy and eggs and checking what the reactions would be in Cycle 2. You should check to see if you have any reactions to them and evaluate how you will treat those foods in your lifetime diet in Cycle 3.

For the foods that you have no intolerances to, you can reintroduce them into your diet without problems. For foods that continue to cause reactions, you can avoid them from your diet completely or check your intolerances to them from time to time.

After many years eating some of the offending foods, your body will be used to these foods. You will look and feel better when you eliminate them from your diet but you should not despair when you develop cravings or withdrawal symptoms. You should continue to follow the Virgin Diet which will help you to overcome the cravings and withdrawal symptoms after some time, so never ever give up.

The best foods to eat
The foods recommended in this book are foods which are grown and raised naturally and humanely which include:

- Organic foods grown without use of pesticides and herbicides
- Unprocessed foods free from additives, preservatives, colorings and flavorings
- Grass-fed beef, lamb and pork
- Free-range chicken and turkey, eggs and ghee
- Pasture-fed wild game
- Non-GMO foods

It also recommends you to eat 1-2 meals each day in the form of Virgin Diet Shakes. Some people eat shakes in the morning and they consume main meals for lunch and supper. There are Virgin Diet Bars which you can take as snacks or as quick meals. The Virgin Diet All-in-One Shake consists of all the nutrients that the body needs.

Food Reactions
There has been a lot of confusion about the terms food intolerance, food allergy and food sensitivity, so we will explain each one of them so that it becomes clear to you right from the start.

Food Intolerance
Food intolerance happens when a specific enzyme that is necessary for digesting a food is absent in your body causing lactose intolerance or gluten intolerance. Food intolerance causes stress to your system and it gives you some of the negative symptoms which include weight gain.

There are some people who have food reactions and cannot tolerate certain types of foods such as gluten or lactose. When they consume these foods, they develop negative responses immediately while others develop negative responses much later.

The symptoms of FI may include gastrointestinal problems, diarrhea, gas, constipation, weight gain and rashes, among others which are usually not life-threatening. The symptoms don't appear immediately after consuming the food in many instances but after hours or days. However, if you continue to consume the same foods time and again, these reactions become chronic.

These food intolerances happen because these people lack a certain chemical or enzyme that is necessary for metabolizing and digesting that specific food. Many people may not understand why this is happening to them and not to others. They need to understand that this is a genetic problem.

Our genes determine who we are and there is nothing we can do except to avoid these foods which we cannot tolerate. These foods cause a reaction which the body uses to mobilize what is known as immunoglobulin G or IgG. This antibody is different from the antibody mobilized by allergic reactions known as immunoglobulin E or IgE. That is why the symptoms of food intolerance are different from those caused by food allergies.

Food Allergy
Food allergy is a specific immune response to a certain food protein. When you have food allergy, your immune system responds when it is exposed to the protein by producing an immunoglobulin known as IgE.

The body then releases natural histamines to deal with the allergy which cause symptoms such as wheezing, itching, hives, breathing problems and digestion problems. In some people, food allergies can cause such severe symptoms or even life-threatening reactions like anaphylaxis.

Food allergy affects the immune system and the reactions occur immediately after consuming certain foods. The allergic reaction takes place even when tiny amounts of allergy causing foods (and drinks) are consumed. This can trigger symptoms within the digestive system but should not be confused with FI symptoms.

It is easy to confuse food allergies with food intolerance. Food intolerance does not affect the immune system like food allergy so the symptoms are not severe.

The majority of the population believes that, they suffer from food allergies but only a small fraction about 6-8% of children and 3-5% of adults do. Most people have food intolerances not food allergies. Some children outgrow these allergic reactions as they grow.

Food Sensitivity
Many of us have food sensitivities which affect us. When you have food sensitivity to a certain food, you react to that food when you consume it. Food sensitivity is a negative reaction to certain foods which may cause heartburn, nausea or cramps after consuming that food. Surprisingly, you may not always get the same symptoms all the time.

The 7 food groups that the Virgin Diet eliminates are likely to cause food intolerance in many people. If you have these reactions to any of these foods, eliminating it from your diet is the best way to boost your metabolism. This will certainly help you to lose weight and maintain a healthy lifestyle. If you notice that you have any food intolerance, stop eating that food immediately.

2: Food Intolerance

Food intolerance (FI) is known medically as non-allergic food hypersensitivity. Food intolerance can be a reaction to food, beverage, preservatives, colorings, flavorings and other food additives which are added to processed foods. This is due to the compounds found in these foods which produce symptoms in the body. However, food intolerance is different from food allergy as we have seen in Chapter 1.

Food intolerance is at times referred to as food allergy. No wonder one-third of the population thinks that they have food allergies but most of them have food intolerance. The difference between the two is that food intolerance involves the digestive system while food allergy involves the immune system.

For a food allergy to occur it requires the presence of immunoglobulin E IgE immune mechanisms or antibodies against that particular food you are allergic to, while food intolerance requires G IgG antibodies. You may ask, what is food intolerance then? Food intolerance or food hypersensitivity happens when you have difficulty digesting a particular food such as gluten, dairy, corn, eggs, soy, peanuts, sugar and sweeteners. Take for example lactose intolerance, when you drink milk or consume other dairy products, this can lead to abdominal pain, gas, diarrhea and constipation. When you have food allergy, even a trace amount of the food you are allergic to, has the potential to cause serious reactions immediately after consuming the food.

Food Intolerance classification
Food intolerances can be classified depending on what causes them.

FI can be caused by:

- Some chemicals or enzymes which the body requires to digest the food substances are absent in lactose intolerance and hereditary fructose intolerance.
- An abnormality in your body which makes it unable to absorb certain nutrients such as fructose.

Non-allergic food hypersensitivity or FI can be difficult to determine because reactions to food substances that are not tolerated can at times be delayed. In addition, a particular food compound that is causing reactions may be present in many different foods. The reaction may also be caused by medications like aspirin derived from plant chemicals.

FI is a non-allergic food hypersensitivity which should not be confused with food allergies. Food intolerance reactions include metabolic, pharmacological and gastro-intestinal responses to certain types of foods or food compounds.

Metabolic food reactions
Metabolic food reactions can be inborn or due to errors of metabolism of the nutrients.

Gastro-intestinal reactions
Gastro-intestinal reactions can be due to mal-absorption or other gastro-intestinal tract abnormalities.

Pharmacological reactions
Pharmacological reactions are caused by natural compound like salicylates or by food additives in form of preservatives, coloring, flavorings and taste enhancers. The chemicals used can cause biochemical or drug-like side effects in some people.

Immunological responses
Immunological responses are when the immune system recognizes certain foods as foreign bodies and starts attacking them.

Psychological reactions

Psychological reactions to the symptoms are caused not by the food itself, but by emotions associated with food.

Toxic food reactions
Toxic food reactions are caused by toxins in the food or substance consumed. The toxins may be present in the food naturally or be caused by a bacteria in the food, or by contamination of food.

Signs and symptoms of food intolerance
The way the food intolerance signs and symptoms present themselves makes them difficult to diagnose than those related to food allergies. The symptoms of food intolerance can be easily mistaken as food allergy. While it is easy to notice when you have food allergies because the symptoms are fast-acting on the immune system, it is not easy to know the "offending foods" in FI responses unless you eliminate and reintroduce them as recommended in this Virgin Diet.

The immunoglobulin IgE responses caused by food allergies are usually fast and acute so it would be hard not to notice them. On the other hand, it can be quite difficult to determine the offending food which is causing food intolerance. This is because offending food generally takes longer to be noticed over a prolonged period of time.

The responses or reactions begin about half an hour after you have consumed the food to 48 hours. Some of the cause and effects like weight gain are quiet natural that so you may never relate them with the FI responses. That is why the Virgin Diet makes a break-through into weight-loss because it points out what has gone wrong and shows you how to rectify it.

Some of the symptoms of food intolerance affect your weight, the skin, the respiratory tract and the gastrointestinal tract.

Skin
Symptoms include skin rashes, hives, eczema, dermatitis and angioedema

Respiratory tract symptoms
Symptoms include asthma, cough, nasal congestion, sinusitis and pharyngeal irritation

Gastro intestinal tract symptoms
Symptoms include nausea, constipation, gas, diarrhea, mouth ulcers, abdominal cramps, irritable bowel syndrome and in the worst cases anaphylaxis.

Food intolerance has been associated with other conditions which include eczema, inflammatory bowel syndrome, irritable bowel syndrome, chronic hepatitis C infection, chronic constipation, NSAID intolerance, ENT problems and functional dyspepsia among other problems.

Causes of FI

Food intolerances are reactions to chemical components of our everyday diet which are more common than food allergies. These reactions are caused by organic chemicals which are present naturally in a wide variety of foods, especially the 7 food groups comprised of both animal and vegetable foods. It is more present in food additives, preservatives, colorings and flavoring.

Food intolerances are therefore caused by adverse reactions to both natural and artificial food compositions when the ingredients are consumed by sensitive people. However, the degree of sensitivity varies between individuals, and some are more affected than others.

At times, deficiency in the chemical digestive enzymes in the body may also cause food intolerances such as lactose intolerance. This happens when the body is unable to produce sufficient lactase to digest the lactose in dairy products such as in milk. However, even in such cases, the dairy foods which have lower lactose content like cheese may hardly trigger a reaction in some people. Hereditary lactose intolerance is also another carbohydrate intolerance that is present in the genes.

There are times when exclusion of certain foods from the diet does not help to identify the chemical which is responsible for the food intolerance. This is due to the fact that several chemicals may be present in the food that is causing reactions and you may be sensitive to several food chemicals. You may have reactions when the foods containing the triggering chemicals are combined in a diet in substantial quantities that exceed your sensitivity threshold. Those people who have food sensitivities have different sensitivity thresholds. When you are more sensitive you react to even tiny amounts of the trigger-causing substance. If you are less sensitive, you may not even notice.

Management of FI
To manage FI you need to change your diet and follow the Virgin Diet by excluding foods that are causing obvious reactions. For many people this may be enough and they may not need professional assistance. But, for some people, FI may not be obvious. If you are unable to identify the food causing reactions especially or if you have other health problems, in such cases it is advisable to seek help from your health care provider or a dietitian. But for most people, everything works out just fine even when they have the health problems.

Most people report that, Virgin Diet relieves pain, aches and mobility problems caused by other health conditions. FI causes inflammation which is the root cause of many illnesses and diseases. As you identify your food intolerances and avoid them, your whole body responds by overcoming these illnesses and diseases. FI causes low metabolism which leads to accumulation of toxins in the body. As you overcome FI, you boost your metabolism by helping your body to get rid of toxins. That is why you feel better and most of the symptoms disappear when you adopt an elimination diet like Virgin Diet.

However, you need to be aware that, during Cycle 1 known as the elimination period and during reintroduction in Cycle 2, you may have food addictions and withdrawal symptoms if you have consumed these foods for the better part of your life. This has been experienced by quite a few people who may have addictions to common foods they are used to eating.

3: The Virgin Diet Cycles

The Virgin Diet is divided into 3 cycles. You can repeat these cycles until you discover the foods that are best suited for your weight loss.
The Virgin Diet has 3 Cycles being

- Elimination
- Reintroduction
- Lifetime Diet

The 3 Virgin Diet Cycles

Cycle 1 Elimination
Eliminate the 7 food groups from your diet for 3 week or 21 days. These are gluten, dairy, corn, soy, eggs, peanuts, sugar and sweeteners which are known to be highly reactive.

Cycle 2 Reintroduction
Reintroduce the foods you had dropped in Cycle 1 to discover which foods cause food intolerances and which ones can help you to achieve optimal health and your weight management goals. Try to reintroduce one of these seven foods into your diet each week for 4 weeks.

Cycle 3 Lifetime Diet
Come up with a lifetime diet plan and maintain it by learning new strategies from Cycle 1 and 2

which will help you achieve your desired weight and keep you healthy for life.

Note that, dark chocolate without added sugar is allowed.

How the Virgin Diet Works

Cycle 1: Elimination
Cycle 1 is the elimination stage and it takes a period of 3 weeks (21 days). During this time, you should cut out all the 7 food groups known as high-FI foods to avoid food intolerances. Don't eat FI foods. Instead, substitute them with healing foods and healthy supplements during this period. You may have cravings for these foods since your body has been addicted to them for a while, but don't be tempted to fall back. Some people may say they had a "false start" in the beginning, but they overcame these cravings once they realized what these foods were doing to them. You will be surprised at the changes in your body when you eliminate these 7 food groups.

Cycle 2: Reintroduction
Cycle 2 is the reintroduction stage which takes 4 weeks (28 days). In each week for the next 4 weeks, you need to test one healthy high-FI food chosen from the 7 food groups by reintroducing it to your diet. Gluten and soy are potentially unhealthy while eggs and dairy are potentially

healthy. But, each individual is different so you should personalize the program and make it your own. The introduction of foods will be based upon your responses whether positive or negative, to help you determine which foods should stay on your Lifetime Diet and which ones should be avoided altogether. If you still have a negative reaction to a certain food or food group, you should let it go or retest it another time.

Cycle 3: Lifetime Diet

You should avoid corn and corn products, eggs, soy, dairy, peanuts, refined sugar and artificial sweeteners most of the time. You should avoid the foods you have intolerances to 95% of the time allowing yourself a few bites now and then which should be 5% of your diet. After 3-6 months, you should reintroduce those potentially healthy foods such as eggs and dairy, or high-FI foods that you had reactions to in Cycle 2 to see if you still have intolerances to them. Repeat this every year (after 12 months).

Virgin Diet Shakes

The Virgin Diet Shakes are very nutritious. You can make the Virgin Diet Shakes at home by using the following ingredients or buy as pre-made shakes that are used as meal replacements.

- vegan pea and rice protein (or plant protein, pea protein, rice protein and hemp protein)
- fiber blend of chia seeds and hemp seeds
- freshly ground flaxseeds or nut butter
- organic frozen berries
- liquid (water, unsweetened almond milk or even coconut water)
- some extras (optional)

You can buy pea and rice protein powder at Amazon or from other online stores, health food stores, food supplement stores, department stores such as Walmart or Target. You may not always get it as pea and rice protein. It might be labeled as plant protein, pea protein, rice protein and hemp protein. Check the label and look at the ingredients to see what kind a protein is contained in the powder. Never use hemp protein on its own in your shake. To have a variety, rotate your fiber by using flax seeds, chia seeds, hemp seeds or extra fiber. Use water, unsweetened almond milk, cashew milk, unsweetened coconut milk, or coconut water. The vegan pea and rice protein is sugar-free, gluten-free and soy free.

You can also buy the Virgin Diet All-In-One pre-made shake powder from the same sources. The optimal vegan protein powder is free of sugar, gluten, soy, dairy products, wheat, corn protein, yeast, animal products, artificial colorings and flavorings. It contains 14 servings per container and every scoop of the powder provides 17 grams of high-quality and non-GMO vegan protein. This is an excellent protein powder for people who have food intolerance and sensitivity to sugar, gluten, dairy, soy, sweeteners or flavorings.

The pre-made Virgin Diet Shake should have:

- Pea protein, rice protein, and/ or hemp protein
- No sugar or at most 5 grams of sugar or less
- No artificial sweeteners
- No gluten
- No dairy or milk solids, whey, egg or soy but soy lecithin is acceptable
- No sugar alcohols but Stevia is okay
- No malt dextrin
- At least 5 grams or more of fiber

Virgin Diet Shake serving size is 2 scoops of the pre-made Virgin Diet All-In-One Shake.

You may not like the taste or texture of Virgin Diet Shakes. If you don't like the texture try to change the consistency of your shake by adding more liquid (water, almond milk, coconut milk etc.) or less fiber. If you don't like the taste try different protein powders to see which ones you like. You can also add a tablespoon of flaxseed or almond butter and different types of berries such as raspberries, blueberries or blackberries or add half a banana (ripe). The fruits will give the taste you are seeking.

Some people like unsweetened almond milk while others like adding coconut milk or pure drinking water. Try to add unsweetened cocoa powder to your shake. Take warm Virgin Diet Shakes by warming the liquid whether it is almond milk, coconut milk or water before adding it to the other ingredients.

4: What to Eat and Avoid During Elimination

The Elimination period lasts for 3 weeks or 21 days

Foods to Eat During Elimination

Week 1: This is the week you want to skip as many foods as possible. Substitute them with Virgin Diet Shake. Drink 2 Virgin Diet Shakes each day, 1 as a meal and 1 as a snack (optional).

Weeks 2 and 3: These 2 weeks are known as the "healing period". Drink 1 Virgin Diet Shake each day plus 2 meals and a snack (optional) daily. If one shake is not enough for you, take 2 shakes daily but this depends on your individual needs.

There are a few things you should know

- To help you track what you are eating, keep a food journal or log of everything you eat.
- Try to eat a substantial well-balanced breakfast. Aim to achieve about 400-500 calories.
- Although the Virgin Diet is not a no-sugar diet, sugar should be avoided or minimized. Whatever you eat should have no more than 5 grams of sugar.

- You should plan your meals to avoid eating the same foods every day which may cause food intolerances when eaten daily. However, you can drink the shakes every day because they are low-reactive.

Timing your meals

As much as eating the right food is important, timing your meals is also important. Drink your Virgin Diet Shakes within 1 hour after waking up. If you like working out the first thing in the morning, you can take ½ the shake before workout and the other ½ after workout.

Time your meals so that you eat every 4 to 6 hours if you are eating 3 meals a day. You can also take 2 meals a day with an afternoon snack. Ensure that you stop eating about 2 to3 hours before you go to bed to give your digestive system enough time to digest the foods.

Plate proportions

The plate proportions should be about:

- 30% non-starchy vegetables
- 25% proteins (clean lean)
- 25% healthy fats
- 15% high-fiber, low-glycemic carbohydrates
- 5% nuts (except peanuts) and seeds
- Low-glycemic fruits

- Fiber
- Drinking water and beverages

Non-starchy vegetables (30%)

Vegetables are rich in antioxidants, vitamins, minerals, fiber and
phytochemicals, so the more you take the better. They will also make you feel full for a longer time because of the fiber.

Non-starchy vegetables - include Alfalfa sprouts, Amaranth, Artichokes, Arugula, Asparagus, Bamboo shoots, Bean sprouts, Beet greens, Bell peppers, Broccoli, Brussels sprouts, Cabbage, Cauliflower, Celery, Chicory, Chives, Collard greens, Coriander, Cucumber, Dandelion greens, Eggplant, Endive, Fennel, Green beans, Green onions, Jalapeño peppers, Kale, Leeks, Lettuce, Mushrooms, Mustard greens, Onions, red and orange Peppers, Radishes, Rhubarb, Pea pods, Shallots, Spinach, Squash (spaghetti and summer), Swiss chard, Tomatoes, Turnip greens, Watercress and Zucchini.

Herbs include - Basil, Cilantro, Garlic, Mint, Parsley, Rosemary, Thyme etc.

(Note that the nightshades i.e. Eggplants, Bell peppers, Jalapeno peppers and Tomatoes may cause issues for some people with arthritis but not all).

Clean lean proteins (25%)

The recommended clean lean proteins in each meal should be 4 to 6 ounces for women and 6 to 8 ounces for men.

Clean lean proteins - include pea-rice protein, quinoa, nuts and seeds, the grass-fed beef, free-range chicken and turkey which are hormone-free, the pasture-fed lamb and pork, wild cold-water fish and wild game.

You can enjoy lean red meat either 3 or 4 times each week. Your main focus should be on wild game and lamb which feed on pasture and then get the rest of your clean lean protein from Virgin Diet Shakes, free-range chicken, turkey, and the lowest-mercury fish.

You can enjoy 6 oz servings of fish 2 or 3 times a week.
The lowest-mercury fish include the Anchovies, the Butterfish, Calamari, Catfish, Clams, King crab, Crawfish, Flounder, Alaskan halibut, Herring, Spiny/rock lobster, Oysters, Pollock, Salmon, Sardines, Scallops, Shrimp, Sole, Tilapia, Trout (freshwater) and Whitefish.

For vegetarians - eat plenty of Nuts, Seeds, Whole grains and Legumes, especially Lentils which are high in protein and Avocadoes.

Healthy fats (25%)

Take 1 to 3 servings of healthy fats per meal. 1 serving is approximately 100 calories. Use 1 tablespoon of healthy fat or 1/3 avocado.
The sources of healthy fats include - Extra-Virgin Olive oil (cook the oil at low heat), Olives, Avocado, Coconut milk or oil, Palm fruit oil, Sesame oil and Wild cold-water fish.

Extra-virgin oil should be cooked on low heat. If you want to use medium or high heat and if you want to fry your food, then use regular olive oil.

High-fiber, low-glycemic carbohydrates (15%)

You should take 15% of your diet in form of high-fiber, low-glycemic vegetables which is about ½ a cup for women and 1 cup for men in each meal.

The carbohydrate in high-fiber low-glycemic foods is released into your system slowly. This helps to stabilize your blood sugar or glucose levels by keeping it low and making you feel fuller for longer periods between meals. As a result, you don't reach out for snacks between meal times and this has a positive effect on weight-loss and insulin levels. These high-fiber low-glycemic foods help to maintain your weight, lower your risk of heart disease and diabetes and improve cholesterol levels. Fiber is not absorbed by the body so it provides roughage to keep your bowels healthy. If you don't consume enough fiber in your diet, you can have constipation.

High-fiber, low glycemic foods include:

- **Legumes** - Adzuki beans, black beans, chick peas, cow peas, great northern beans, kidney beans, lentils, lima beans, mung beans, navy beans, split peas and white beans. Whenever it will be possible, consume organic, soaked, sprouted or fermented lentils, beans and peas since they have the highest nutrient content.

- **Whole non-gluten grains** - Brown rice, Brown rice pasta or Quinoa pasta, Brown rice wraps, Millet, Oat bran and Quinoa (soaked, sprouted, or fermented).

- **Starchy vegetables** - Beets, Butternut Squash, Carrots (raw), Corn, French beans, Green Peas, Okra, Parsnips, Plantain, Pumpkin, Sweet Potatoes, Winter Squash and Yams. Avoid eating potatoes because they have a high glycemic index.

Whole non-gluten grains, legumes, and starchy vegetables can be included in your Virgin Diet but should not be eaten in excess. Take 1 to 4 servings a day, assuming that 1 serving is about ½ a cup.

Nuts and Seeds (5%)

Take 1 to 3 servings of nuts and seeds each day. This includes raw Nuts (except peanuts) and Nut Butter. The nuts include Almonds, Cashews, Hazelnuts and Walnuts or 1 Tablespoon of Nut Butter (except Peanut Butter). You can take ghee from grass-fed cows as it has no milk solids. Raw seeds include Chia, Hemp and freshly ground Flaxseed.

Soak the nuts overnight to lower the effects of lectins, phytates and any other enzyme inhibitors.

Low-glycemic fruits
Low-glycemic fruits are the best and they include - Blackberries, Blueberries, Elderberries, Gooseberries, Raspberries and Strawberries. Moderate-glycemic fruits which you should eat in moderation include Apples, Apricots, Cherries, Grapefruits, Kiwi, Lemons, Limes, Melons, Oranges, Passion Fruits, Peaches, Pears, Plums, Pomegranates and Tangerines.

Fiber

You should consume a minimum of 50 grams of fiber daily and keep increasing your fiber intake as your body adjusts to it. Soluble fiber is good for you.

The top sources of fiber include:

- Lentils
- Nuts i.e. Almonds, Cashews, Hazelnuts and Walnuts etc.
- Seeds i.e. Chia seeds and freshly ground Flaxseeds etc.
- Vegetables i.e. Avocado, Broccoli, Eggplants, Kale and Winter squash etc.
- Fruits i.e. Apples, Blackberries, Blueberries, Raspberries and Strawberries etc.
- Whole grains i.e. Quinoa, millet etc.

Water and other healthy beverages
Pure drinking water, green vegetable juice and green tea are good options. Green vegetable juices and smoothies should be prepared with low-glycemic green vegetables such as cabbage, celery, kale, broccoli and spinach. Don't add high-glycemic fruits or vegetables such as beets, apples, carrots and okra which should be avoided or minimized. Powdered green drinks are okay as long as they are sugar-free.

- *Daily total* - The daily total intake of water and healthy beverages should be 64 ounces at minimum. If you are heavy, you exercise heavily, or if you live in hot climates, the intake should be more than that.
- *Morning* - Drink 16 ounces when you get up in the morning
- *Before meals* – Drink 16 ounces 30 to 60 minutes before meals.
- *During meals* - During meal times take 4 to 8 ounces in every meal.
- *After meals* - Drink water or beverages again 60 minutes after meals.
- *Before bedtime* - 8 ounces

Limit your coffee intake to 1 or 2 cups per day especially organic coffee.

Alternative Sweeteners

Many artificial sweeteners used in foods like aspartame could lead to weight gain, cravings and diabetes. There are safer alternative sweeteners which you could use. These include:

- Stevia - 100% organic pure Stevia extract which has no malt dextrin
- Monk fruit sweetener
- Erythritol
- Xylitol

Healing Foods and Spices

There are several healing foods you should add to your Virgin Diet. Aloe Vera juice, Apples, Avocado, Beets, Berries, Broccoli, Cabbage, Chia seeds, Cilantro, Cinnamon, Coconut and Coconut Milk, Dandelion greens, Extra-Virgin Olive oil, Flaxseed, Garlic, Ginger, Green tea, Lentils, Palm Fruit Oil, Pomegranate, Red Onions, Red Peppers, Rosemary, Seafood (including Salmon, Sardines and Scallops), Sweet Potato, Turmeric and other healing foods such as Artichokes, Oregano Sauerkraut, Sea salt and Xylitol.

During the elimination period it is helpful to eat soaked, fermented, and sprouted foods and also pickled foods. Note that this does not mean commercially pickled foods. These are prepared traditionally like the Sauerkraut and Kimchi. You can also have Kombucha as long as no sugar has been added. Fermented fish sauces are also great but they should be gluten-free. There are also some Dark chocolate brands which don't have dairy and are gluten-free.

B. Foods to Avoid During Elimination

Virgin Diet Cycle 1 What You Should Not Eat

Avoid eating the top 7 high-FI foods completely during elimination.

1. *Gluten*

Gluten is found in Alcoholic drinks (some), Baked beans, Biscuits, Blue cheese, Bran (all types), Bread, Breadcrumbs, Bread rolls, Breakfast cereals (some), Brown rice syrup, Bulgur wheat, Cakes, Chocolate (some brands), Chutneys, Cookies, Crisp breads, Gravy powders, Hydrolyzed vegetable protein (HVP), Licorice, Malt vinegar, Malted drinks, many Salad dressings, Matzo flour, Meat and Fish pastes, Muesli, Muffins, Mustard powder, Pancakes, Pasta (i.e. macaroni and spaghetti), Pastry, Pickles, Pie crust, Pizza, Pretzels, Pringles potato chips, Rye bread, Sauces (because they are usually thickened with flour), Sausages (rusk), Scones, Semolina, Soups (with roux), Soy sauce, Spice blends, Stock cubes, Stuffing, Waffles and White pepper.

2. *Dairy*

Dairy consists of Butter (and many types of margarines), Chocolate (except some of the dark chocolate types), Cottage cheese, Milk and Yogurts (cow's, goat's and sheep's), Cheeses, Cream, Cream (sour, whipped), Cream soups (and chowders), Creamy cheese or Butter sauces (served on vegetables and meats), Creamy soups and sauces, Ice cream, Baked products with dairy ingredients (Bread, Cakes, Cookies, Crackers, Desserts, Muffins), Baking mixes and Pancake mix (many), many Canned foods (soups, spaghetti, ravioli), many Salad dressings (ranch, blue cheese, creamy), Mashed potatoes (with milk, butter or margarines), Shakes and Hot chocolate drinks and powders as well as whey protein powder.

Many times dairy is listed on labels as Butter, Butter flavor, Buttermilk or Buttermilk solids, Casein, cream, cream cheese, cottage cheese, Lactose, milk solids, non-fat milk solids, whey or yogurt.

3. *Eggs*

You should avoid consumption of eggs from corn or soy-fed animals which are fed on GMOs. Eggs are also found in baked products, batter mixes, Bavarian cream, boiled dressing, breads, cake flours, cream fillings, custards, egg drop soup, egg beaters, French toast, Fritters, frosting, Ice cream, malted drinks, mayonnaise, meat loaf, noodles, pancakes, puddings, salad dressings, sauces, sausages, tartar sauce and waffles.

The Egg may at times be printed on labels as Albumin, egg protein, egg white, egg yolk, globulin, ovalbumin, powdered egg and vitelline, among other names.

4. *Corn*

Avoid consumption of corn commonly found in many Breakfast cereals, corn chips, corn syrup, dextrose, glucose, high fructose corn syrup, maize, margarine, popcorns, corn starch, corn oil and vegetable oil.

5. *Soy*
Soy is usually found in energy bars, energy shakes, pre-made foods, soy beans, soy protein powders, soy milk, soy sauce, tempeh, tofu and veggie burgers

6. *Peanuts*
Avoid eating peanuts as well as consuming those peanuts found in baked products, baking mixes, biscuits, Breakfast cereals, candy, chili sauce, Chinese dishes, cookies, egg rolls, Ice cream, margarines, milk formula, pastry, Peanut butter, Thai dishes, Vegetable fat and oil. These products may alternatively be listed on labels as Emulsifier, Flavoring, Groundnut and Peanut or Peanut butter.

7. *Sugar and Artificial sweeteners*

Sugar is found in many products including:

- Agave nectar
- Barley malt
- Beet sugar
- Blackstrap molasses
- Brown sugar
- Cane juice and Cane sugar
- Castor sugar
- Confectioner's sugar

- Corn sweeteners
- Corn syrup
- Date sugar
- Dextrin
- Dextrose
- Fructose
- Fruit juice (sweetened)
- Fruit juice concentrates
- Glucose
- Glucose solids
- Golden sugar
- Golden syrup
- Grape sugar
- High fructose corn syrup
- Honey
- Icing sugar
- Lactose
- Malt syrup
- Malt dextrin
- Maltose
- Maple syrup
- Molasses
- Raw sugar
- Rice syrup
- Sorbitol
- Sorghum syrup
- Sucrose
- Sugar
- Syrup

- Yellow sugar

Artificial sweeteners are part of the ingredients used in the manufacture of Diet sodas and other sweetened foods. Some of the sweeteners used include Acesulfame potassium, Alitame, Aspartame, Aspartame-acesulfame salt, Cyclamate, NutraSweet, Saccharin, Splenda and Sucralose.

The Virgin diet is not a no-sugar diet, but it is a low-glycemic diet so you should not take sugars and sweeteners which have a high glycemic index GI. Whatever you eat should not have more than 5 grams of sugar.

Avoid the following foods:

- Processed foods - Avoid processed foods, including even gluten-free processed foods.

- GMOs - Genetically modified foods (GMOs).

- Proteins from - commercially raised animals fed on corn and soy grains and those given hormones.

- Farm-raised fish - that is heavy in mercury and other heavy metals. These include King mackerel, Marlin, Shark and Swordfish among others.

- Fats - avoid refined, rancid and hydrogenated trans-fats and saturated fats.

- Nightshades - Eggplants, Peppers, Potatoes and Tomatoes can cause problems for those with joint pain.
- High-glycemic index GI foods – fruits such as Bananas, Grapes, Mango, Papaya, Pineapple and Watermelon, Fruit juices, Dried fruits, Potatoes and any other high-glycemic index foods.
- Beverages - Soft drinks, Alcohol and Drinking water in plastic bottles.

Limit your intake of Saltwater bass, Bluefish, Atlantic halibut, Maine lobster, Sea trout, Fresh blue-fin tuna, Cod, Crab, Monkfish and Fresh Pacific albacore tuna.

5: Foods to Eat and Avoid During Reintroduction

This Cycle 2 lasts 4 weeks or 28 days. You should test one potentially healthy food every week for at least 4 weeks. These are high food intolerance or FI foods. Check your reactions so you will know whether that food will stay in your diet or not.

Foods to Eat During Reintroduction

Try to reintroduce one food per week which you had eliminated in Cycle 1. In Virgin Diet, eggs and dairy are known to be potentially healthy while soy and gluten are potentially unhealthy. However, you should reintroduce them to test whether you need to eliminate them in your diet completely. But one thing you should be careful about is to use only healthy and unprocessed foods. Don't fall back to unhealthy foods and processed foods if you want to lose weight permanently. The foods you are reintroducing should be taken in moderate amounts. Do not indulge in these foods during reintroduction.

Week 1: Reintroduce Soy to your diet

From Monday to Thursday of Week 1, add soy beans or soy products to 1 meal each day.

From Friday to Sunday, take your soy-free diet again and keep a journal of your symptoms every day with and without soy. Track your food reactions (if any) every day of the week. You should also take at least one Virgin Diet Shake every day of the week, take plenty of pure drinking water and healthy beverages to stay hydrated and time your meals as recommended.

Week 2: Reintroduce Gluten to your diet
From Monday to Thursday of Week 2, add gluten to 1 meal each day.

From Friday to Sunday, take your gluten-free diet again and keep a journal of your symptoms every day with and without gluten. Track your food reactions (if any) every day of the week and write them down. You should also take at least one Virgin Diet Shake every day of the week, take plenty of pure drinking water and healthy beverages to stay hydrated and time your meals as recommended.

Week 3: Reintroduce Eggs to your diet
From Monday to Thursday of Week 1, add eggs or egg products to 1 meal each day in that week.

From Friday to Sunday, take your egg-free diet again and keep a journal of your symptoms every day with and without the eggs. Track your food reactions (if any) every day of the week. You should also take at least one Virgin Diet Shake every day of the week, take plenty of pure drinking water and healthy beverages to stay hydrated and time your meals as recommended.

Week 4: Reintroduce Dairy to your diet
From Monday to Thursday of Week 1, add dairy or daily products to 1 meal each day.

From Friday to Sunday, take your dairy-free diet again and keep a journal of your symptoms every day with and without dairy. Track your food reactions (if any) every day of the week. You should also take at least one Virgin Diet Shake every day of the week, take plenty of pure drinking water and healthy beverages to stay hydrated and time your meals as recommended.

If you cannot tolerate cow's milk, you should try goat's milk and sheep's milk in this Cycle 2 to see which one works for you. Consume the milk raw and fermented in form of kefir or yogurt and see whether you will tolerate it.

The Virgin Diet helps you to lose weight and become healthy by eliminating foods that you cannot tolerate. You may discover that, you can tolerate soy, gluten or eggs in this reintroduction cycle but we recommend that you don't add these foods back to your diet in the following 3 weeks. However, if you notice food intolerance on the first day, then you should avoid eating that food. You can recheck your reaction again after 3 months but if you don't want to, you can cancel that food from your diet.

If you notice that you have reaction on the fourth day of the week, you can then add that food to your diet, not daily but every fourth day. If you take it more often than that, you might notice that you react to it more intensely. If you notice no reaction, especially to eggs or dairy which are regarded as potentially healthy, then you can take these foods every 2-3 days but not every day.

B. What not to Eat during Reintroduction

Apply the foods that you avoided in Cycle 1 as you reintroduce the foods to eat as listed in Cycle 2

6: How to Choose Your Lifetime Diet

The diet that you end up with in Cycle 3 should be your lifetime diet. You should stick to this diet to help you lose weight permanently and maintain a healthy body.

A. What you should eat during your Lifetime Diet

You should start eating the foods in Cycle 1 again as you add the foods that you have been able to tolerate which you tested in Cycle 2.

You should adhere to the Virgin Diet plate proportions as you stick to non-starchy vegetables, clean lean proteins, healthy fats, high-fiber low-glycemic carbohydrates, nuts and seeds, and plenty of pure drinking water.

Avoid sugar and artificial sweeteners, gluten, corn, soy, eggs and peanuts if you reacted to them. Include healthy eggs and dairy in your diet if you did not react to them in Cycle 2 when you reintroduced them. In such cases you can eat them normally every other day but not every day. If you had a reaction say on the fourth day of the week, you can eat them after 4 days.

If you had immediate reactions you should avoid them for at least 3 months and then retest them. If you get reactions again, you can forget them for the time being or keep retesting every few months or cancel them from your lifetime diet.

In addition to the above, you should follow the meal timing, substitute 1 meal every day with a Virgin Diet Shake or All-in-One Shake, keep your body hydrated and use non-food rewards to reward yourself for achieving the milestones you have set.

Low Intolerance (Low-LI) Foods
The following are some low-FI foods which are the least reactive foods in the Virgin Diet which you should include in your lifetime diet.

- *Proteins* - Free-range chicken and turkey, pasture-fed lamb, pork and wild game, pea, rice or hemp protein and wild cold-water fish, nuts, sees etc.
- *Non-starchy vegetables*: Broccoli, cabbage, cauliflower, deep green leafy vegetables, kale, spinach etc.
- *Fruit*: Apples, blueberries, raspberries, blackberries etc.
- *Fats*: Avocado, chia seeds, coconut oil and coconut milk, extra-virgin olive oil, freshly ground flaxseed meal, and palm fruit oil.
- *High-fiber starchy carbs*: Brown rice, lentils, quinoa, sweet potatoes etc.

The foods should be hormone-free foods with no additives, preservatives, colorings and flavorings and raised or grown with no pesticides and herbicides. Take organically grown foods.

If by now you still want to lose more weight follow these guidelines:

- Replace 2 meals daily with Virgin Diet Shakes
- Replace high-fiber starchy carbohydrates with plenty of non-starchy vegetables which are low in calories
- Drink plenty of green juices, smoothies and green tea which will boost your metabolism
- Add more fiber to your diet to provide roughage.
- Drink plenty of water
- Substitute high fat animal proteins (i.e. as grass-fed beef and lamb) with low fat ones (i.e. chicken breasts, turkey breasts)

Food intolerances keep changing so you should repeat Cycles 1, 2, and 3 every year. Keep repeating this in your lifetime to see what you can tolerate from time to time and what you cannot.

B. Foods to avoid during your Lifetime Diet

You should not eat the foods listed in Cycle 2 in addition to any foods you have reacted to. Avoid the forbidden foods that you have not reacted to negatively which have been listed among foods you should never eat. Even if you have not reacted to these foods, you know they are not good for you. Some reactions are not noticeable. You only notice what you are going through when you become overweight or when you fall sick.

Avoid the following offending foods in your diet:

- GMOs - Genetically modified foods (GMOs) should be avoided.

- All processed foods - since they are loaded with refined sugar, preservatives, colorings, flavorings and other additives to appeal to our taste buds. Avoid these foods and take natural foods rich in antioxidants, vitamins, minerals, fiber and other nutrients.

- Beef, chicken, turkey, pork and lamb – from animals fed on corn and soy grains which are usually GMOs and animals given hormones, antibiotics and artificial treatments which leave traces of dioxin which is not good for your health.

- Heavy-mercury fish - are usually farm-raised fish and other fish such as some types of

Salmon and Tuna, King mackerel, Marlin, Shark and Swordfish among others.

- Fats – avoid 'bad fats' which are high in LDC cholesterol such as refined, rancid and hydrogenated trans-fats and saturated fats.

- High-glycemic index GI foods – of all types i.e. fruits such as Bananas, Grapes, Mango, Papaya, Pineapple and Watermelon, Fruit juices, Dried fruits i.e. Raisins, Dates, Figs etc., Potatoes and any other high-glycemic index foods.

- Beverages - Soft drinks since they are loaded with refined sugar and colorings, fruit juices loaded with artificial sweeteners and drinking water sold in plastic bottles.

Health benefits of Virgin Diet

The Virgin Diet has many benefits in addition to weight loss. Some of the benefits include: relieve from abdominal cramps, acne, ADHD, anxiety, arthritis (osteoarthritis and rheumatoid arthritis), asthma, bloating, blood sugar spikes, candida (or yeast overgrowth), chronic stuffy nose, congestion, constipation, depression, diarrhea, eczema, fatigue, food addictions, food cravings, food intolerance and sensitivity, gas, headaches, heartburn, hyperactivity, inability to lose weight, insomnia, insulin resistance, irritable bowel syndrome, irritable bowel disorder, joint pains, moodiness, muscle pain and aches, obesity, low energy levels, psoriasis, sinusitis, skin rashes, small intestinal bacterial overgrowth and many other problems.

Those who have followed the Virgin Diet have reported that it alleviated many symptoms such as inflammation, swelling, on ankles and other areas, fatigue, post exercise exhaustion, chronic muscle pains, and it lowers high blood pressure and cholesterol levels. Some have reported it has led to increased energy, joint mobility, increased flexibility and increased range of motion for arthritis patients and less stress. Most people feel more healthy and vibrant and they enjoy walking and other activities they were unable to do previously.

In Cycle 2 you will know what drags you down and what pulls you up. Ultimately eat what works best for you.

7: How to Lose Weight and Maintain a Healthy Lifestyle

Some people may have a problem when starting on the Virgin Diet because they have to drop most of the foods they have been used to, but losing those unwanted pounds is a great incentive for them. The Virgin Diet is a success because once you discover your food intolerances, things fall in place. It nourishes your body to make you look and feel better as you lose weight quickly. When you start taking this diet seriously, you will lose weight permanently, become healthier in all spheres of your life and maintain a healthy lifestyle for the rest of your life.

How food intolerance can affect you
There are many foods you may be eating right now that could be triggering your food intolerances. These include soy products, whole grain bread because of gluten, egg-whites because of eggs and Greek yogurt because of dairy. Your body may be unable to tolerate these foods which may cause inability to lose weight.

An inflammatory diet composed of the offending foods causes inflammation to your body tissue which is the root cause of many illnesses and diseases. Your body cells are deprived of oxygen and they become sick while metabolism is impaired. The only way you can overcome these problems is to follow the Virgin Diet which will help you to identify the foods in your diet causing food intolerances.

How do I find out if I have food intolerances?
You may visit a health care practitioner for an IgG test that shows some of the most common food sensitivities you could be having. But this examination may not show all the hormonal and genetic food intolerances.

The best way to do this is to test the foods yourself as recommended in this Virgin Diet. This involves testing your own body by eliminating the high-FI (food intolerant) foods for 3 weeks in Cycle 1 followed by reintroduction of these foods one by one within 4 weeks in Cycle 2 as we have discussed earlier. When you challenge your body of what it can or cannot tolerate by adding the foods back into your diet one by one, you will know how you feel and come up with your lifetime diet. However, you can retest these foods if you want to.

Food intolerances are more chronic
Many of the symptoms such as weight gain and obesity caused by food intolerances slowly slip in while making you feel normal after consuming these foods, unlike when you have food allergies. You may therefore not make an obvious connection

between the foods you eat or drink and the symptoms they create because of delayed reactions. That is why you need to adopt the Virgin Diet to know the foods you should avoid, in order to lose weight and maintain a healthy lifestyle.

The most common symptoms

Some of the most common symptoms of food intolerance which you will be able to overcome with the Virgin diet include:

- weight gain and inability to lose weight
- gas
- indigestion
- bloating
- fatigue
- mental fog
- irritability
- mood swings

If you are eating foods that your body cannot tolerate, you will likely gain weight and look much older than your actual age. Everyone should be able to benefit from dropping these 7 highly reactive foods for 3 weeks or 21 days. The diet plan can be tried by anyone who is concerned about his or her overall health. It helps to detoxify the body and provide it with nutrients that it needs.

Virgin Diet Bars

The Virgin Diet Bars contain non-GMO ingredients and the ingredients like cashew butter, rice protein, chia seeds, cacao and vegetable glycerin are organic. These bars don't have artificial sweeteners and preservatives.

The Virgin Diet Bars are meant to be a healthy snack, an emergency meal when you don't have time to prepare a meal, or as a satisfying dessert without added sugar that most desserts have. They are good to take during any cycle of the Virgin Diet. You may only need half a bar as a snack and a whole bar for a mini-meal or emergency food.

The Virgin Diet Bar is sourced from organic cashew butter, which is a rich source of healthy fat referred to as "good fat" (monounsaturated fat). For a long time, fat was labeled as bad, but today we know that the body needs healthy fat to function properly.

Many weight-loss programs recommend avoiding fat when losing weight but it is the "bad fat" which should be avoided. Monounsaturated fat is good and the bad fats that you should avoid are trans-fats and saturated fats. The walnuts in the bars and the organic chia seeds provide you with Omega 3 fatty acids which are anti-inflammatory. These are good for your health since food intolerance causes inflammation. The fats in Virgin Diet Bars are healthy, satisfying and have a rich taste.

Soy lecithin

The only form of soy that you should take in the Virgin Diet is soy lecithin. Although soy causes food intolerance which may ultimately lead to weight gain or inability to lose weight, soy lecithin is safe to take. That is why it is used as a common ingredient in many gluten-free vegan shakes and protein bars, among other foods. Soy lecithin is gluten-free and it is the protein in soy that causes food intolerance and allergies but not soy lecithin. It is therefore used in some Virgin Diet Bar as an emulsifier.

Usually, it is the protein component of soy that creates problems and this does not happen when soy lecithin is used because it is a fat, so it does not create negative reactions.

Emulsifiers help mix fat and water together. Soy lecithin transports or delivers the fat-soluble nutrients around the body for optimal absorption. You should read labels carefully to ensure that any food that contains soy lecithin is non-GMO.

The Virgin Diet Bars are free of gluten, soy other than soy lecithin, dairy, eggs, peanuts and artificial sweeteners so they are ideal for weight loss. Soy lecithin is therefore suitable for people who cannot tolerate soy. In addition to its role as an emulsifier, soy lecithin also stabilizes the foods you eat helping powders to blend well in water.

Soy lecithin is suitable for all the 3 cycles of Virgin Diet.

Virgin Diet Shake formulas
The Virgin Diet Shake formulas are available in plant-based and animal-based proteins. There are people who enjoy the plant-based Virgin Diet Shakes while others ask for alternatives. Those who prefer animal-derived protein can get animal-based protein powders that are dairy-free. They are prepared from pasture fed animals that are raised without any hormones or antibiotics. All the Virgin Diet Shake powders recommended in this book are high-quality proteins that are dairy-free, GMO-free and are rich in vitamins, minerals, fiber and other nutrients.

You can use the All-in-One Shakes in Cycles 1, 2, and 3. The All-in-One Shake is an ideal way to get your protein-rich breakfast.

Plate Proportions
When adopting this Virgin Diet, you don't count calories but you should have the right plate proportions.

- 25% of your plate in all meals should contain clean lean protein.
- 25% of healthy fats, there is some good fat in the protein of grass-fed, pasture-fed animals and free-range chicken and turkey. However, vegetarians and vegans should get healthy fat from avocado, coconut, extra-virgin olive oil, nuts and seeds.
- 30% of your meals should be non-starchy leafy and cruciferous vegetables.
- 15% of high-fiber, low-glycemic carbs and 5% nuts and seeds

If your goal is to lose weight, you will exceed those expectations with this Virgin Diet.

The Virgin Diet focuses on food intolerances while most weight-loss programs focus on workouts and diets that may not work for you. You may be doing everything right in the weight-loss regimen you have chosen and still fail to lose weight.

When you eliminate the 7 food groups and avoid foods that trigger food intolerances you lose weight fast within a few weeks. It is important to know your body, what it wants and what it does not want. Why? Food intolerances may be the ones holding you back. In fact, they may sabotage your health and hold your weight, even making you to gain more weight despite eating "healthy foods". In most instances, weight comes off fast while the gas, constipation, bloating and fatigue go away. The aches that come with food intolerance disappear and you start feeling good again.

Sugar

Consuming more sugar is linked with weight gain. Sugar and other high glycemic foods like potatoes are linked with weight gain and other health conditions like Type 2 diabetes. This is due to the fact that after consuming them, the blood glucose level rises and the body produce more insulin to fight them. Excess insulin in the body leads to weight gain because the liver is not able to metabolize the foods effectively. Lessening the sugar in your diet helps in reducing weight and obesity.

The "hidden sugars" in many products can sabotage your weight-loss and also your health so you should read the labels carefully. You should also be aware that some common foods we eat on a daily basis are loaded with sugar or artificial sweeteners. These include cakes, biscuits, muffins, soft drinks etc. It is not just the sugar you add to your coffee or tea that matters.
Raisins, dates and figs fall in the high-sugar fruits category and so you should avoid them especially in Cycle 1. They are in fact concentrated sugar or as you would like to call them "natural candy".

Dark Chocolate
In this diet you are allowed to eat 100% dark chocolate which has no added sugar. The dark chocolate satisfies your sugar cravings if you have a sweet tooth or you can take high-cocoa brands with no more than 5 grams of sugar.

Ghee
You can substitute ghee for butter or take grass-fed animal butter. The casein found in most common butter brands cause dairy intolerances you want to avoid if you are dairy intolerant.

Coconut milk
Coconut milk might not go well with some people and if you have problems with it, you should take coconut water, almond milk or cashew milk.

8: Virgin Diet Recipes

You can create your own recipes from the healthy foods in this book. People have different preferences depending on their taste buds and as long as you choose the right foods recommended in the 3 cycles, you can create delicious meals that you and your family will love.

Vegetable and Berry Protein Smoothie

Serves 1

Ingredients:

- 8 ounces Almond or Coconut Milk, unsweetened
- 1 scoop Raw Protein Powder
- 1 teaspoon Flaxseeds
- 1 cup fresh or frozen Blueberries
- 1 cup fresh or frozen Strawberries
- 1 handful Organic Baby Spinach
- 1 handful Organic Kale, stemmed and chopped

Preparation:

Put the flaxseeds in a blender and process them until they are ground. Add all the other ingredients and pulse until smooth. Serve in a glass and enjoy.

Fruit and Vegetable Protein Smoothie

Serves 2 - 3

Ingredients:

- 2 cups Organic Berries, Blackberries, Blueberries, Raspberries, Strawberries or Marion berries
- 2 cups Coconut Milk or Almond Milk, unsweetened
- 1 cup Organic Baby Spinach
- 1 cup Organic Kale, stemmed and chopped
- 1 Kiwi Fruit, peeled and chopped
- 1 Apple, cored and cut (wedges)
- 1 Orange or Grapefruit, freshly squeezed juice
- ½ cup Organic Dandelion Greens
- ½ cup Vanilla Powder, Non-soy Non whey
- ¼ cup Flaxseed meal
- 1 teaspoon Chia seed

Preparation:

Put all the ingredients in a blender and puree until smooth. Serve in a glass.

Peach and Raspberry Protein Smoothie

Serves 2

Ingredients:

- 1 scoop Pea Rice Protein Powder, Vanilla

- 1 cup frozen Peaches
- ½ cup fresh or frozen Raspberries
- 1 Tablespoon Coconut Milk, unsweetened
- 12 ounces Water
- 1 teaspoon Xylitol
- 2 teaspoons Fiber

Preparation:

Place the coconut milk, raspberries and xylitol in a saucepan and cook on low heat until you make a sauce.

Keep the sauce in the fridge for at least 30 minutes or until you are ready to make the smoothie. Pour the remaining ingredients in a blender and puree until smooth.

Pour the mixture in 2 glasses and mix with the chilled raspberry sauce.
Serve

Strawberry and Chocolate Protein Shake

Serves 1

Ingredients:

- 2 scoops All-in-One Chocolate Protein Powder
- 1 cup Strawberries, frozen (or fresh Strawberries with 4 ice cubes)

- 1 cup Almond Milk
- 1 Tablespoon Almond butter
- 1 Tablespoon Chia seeds, ground

Preparation:

Place all the ingredients in a blender and process until the mixture is smooth. If you are using fresh strawberries, add 4 ice cubes.
Serve in a glass.

Fruit and Nut Oatmeal

Serves 1

Ingredients:

- 1/3 cup Oatmeal, gluten-free
- 1/3 cup Strawberries. Chopped
- 1 Tablespoon Almonds, sliced
- 1 teaspoon Flaxseeds
- 1 splash of Almond Milk, unsweetened

Preparation:

Place the oatmeal, strawberries in a saucepan and add some water. Bring the mixture to a boil and simmer for 10 minutes while stirring regularly.

Remove the oatmeal from the heat and wait for a few minutes for it to thicken.

Put in a serving bowl and add the splash of almond milk.

Stir in the almonds and flaxseeds then serve for breakfast.

Mixed Berries and Flaxseed Pancakes

Serves 2 - 3

Ingredients:

- 2 scoops of All-in-One Shake Mix
- ½ cup Mixed Berries
- 1/3 cup Almond Milk, unsweetened
- 1/3 cup Oatmeal
- 1 Tablespoon Flaxseeds, ground
- 1 Tablespoon Water

Preparation:

Put the flaxseeds in water for 5 minutes.
Mix the other ingredients in a mixing bowl and combine. Add the flaxseeds while stirring the mixture until everything blends together.

Heat a skillet at high-medium heat and pour the mixture into 3 round pancakes. Cook for 2-3 minutes and flip over the other side. Fry for 1-2 minutes and serve.

Chicken and Spinach Main Dish

Serves 2

Ingredients:

- 2 Chicken breasts, boneless and skinned
- 4 cups Spinach, fresh and chopped
- 1 Tablespoon Olive oil
- ¼ cup Onion, chopped
- 1 ½ cup Chicken broth
- 2 Garlic cloves, chopped
- ½ Lemon, freshly squeezed juice

Preparation:

Heat the olive oil on a skillet on medium heat and then add the chicken breasts, half of the chicken broth, onion and garlic. Cover and reduce the heat. Cook until all the broth has evaporated which is approximately 10 minutes.

Add the fresh spinach and the remaining chicken broth. Cover and cook for 3 minutes. Put the food on 2 serving plates and drizzle the lemon juice on top. Serve.

Chicken with Baked Vegetables

Serves 4

Ingredients:

- 1 ½ pound tender Chicken Breasts, boneless and skinless
- 4 Carrots, chopped 1 inch
- 4 cups Arugula
- 1 Broccoli, chopped into florets
- 1 Cauliflower, chopped into florets
- 3 Tablespoons Olive Oil
- 1 Tablespoons Lemon juice, fresh
- 1 teaspoon Thyme, chopped
- 1 teaspoon Rosemary, chopped
- Salt and Pepper to taste

Preparation:

Pre-heat the oven at 425 Degrees F. Arrange the carrots, broccoli and cauliflower on 2 baking sheets. Sprinkle 2 tablespoons olive oil and the lemon juice on top and toss the vegetables.

Roast the vegetables in the oven until lightly brown at approximately 20 minutes.

Mix rosemary, thyme and any other herb you want in a small bowl.

Season the chicken with salt and pepper and then coat it with the herbs.

Heat the remaining oil on a large skillet or saucepan using medium heat.

Place the chicken on the pan and fry until it is cooked (about 5-7 minutes)

Serve the chicken on 4 plates over the arugula with the baked vegetables.

Turkey with Vegetables

Serves 2

Ingredients:

- 1 pound Turkey
- 16 ounce can Beans (black, adzuki or navy), or pre-cooked
- 1 Onion, chopped
- 2 Garlic cloves, minced
- 1 Tablespoon Coconut oil
- 3 cups Greens (kale, beet greens, bok choy or other greens)
- Salt and pepper to taste

Preparation:

Put the coconut oil in a skillet or sauce pan and heat over medium heat. Add the onions and sauté them until they are translucent. Add garlic and stir.

Add the turkey and cook until light brown. Mix in the beans and vegetables and cook until ready. Season with salt and pepper then serve.

Conclusion

Life is about choices. The choices we make determine who we are and what we become. You may choose a career, a spouse, a holiday destination, where to live, what to wear and your pet among other life choices. Your health is your wealth and you need to choose foods that will help you to lose weight and to boost your metabolism so you can live a healthier life.

The Virgin Diet sums it all for you. You may be surprised to learn that some of the most common foods which you consume every day are offending foods. You need to therefore check your food intolerances as recommended.

This book is about eliminating the seven FI foods. After the elimination period of 3 weeks, these foods are reintroduced in the reintroduction stage of 4 weeks to see if they were the ones causing food intolerance.

The Virgin Diet eliminates these 7 food groups and each group consists of several foods. Take for example dairy, the food group includes milk, cheese, yogurt, cream and butter as well as products with these ingredients. These food groups consist of common foods found in many diets. You need to read the food labels carefully to make sure none of the offending foods are included in the foods you are buying.

The Virgin Diet boosts your metabolism which had slowed down because of consuming foods which your body could not tolerate. Your metabolism helps to burn the excess "bad" fat in the body and eliminate toxins that have accumulated in your system. You ultimately become healthier, more energetic and vibrant. Your life changes and you start feeling happy again. You will be able to do the things you are passionate about without tiring easily.

Made in the USA
Middletown, DE
05 July 2016